Tati Helene

Diaphragmatic hypertonia in lyric singers

Tati Helene

Diaphragmatic hypertonia in lyric singers

Causes, consequences and possible approaches

ScienciaScripts

Tati Helene

Diaphragmatic hypertonia in lyric singers

Causes, consequences and possible approaches

Thanks to

To the dearest Angélica Castilho and Cristina Prota, masters and friends, who accepted to orient me in such a new research theme.
To all my fellow singers who inspire me every day to continue researching about us, symbolized in this book by dear Elisabete Almeida, who kindly wrote the preface.
To my dear friends Thayana Roverso and Vinícius Atique, who said yes without blinking to my requests and were the models and photographers for the photos.
To my beloved sister who, in her busy routine, found time to draw for this book.
And to my companion, friend and love, who besides always encouraging me, reviews all my literary adventures.

CONTENT

Preface

Opening paths to the future

When we try to measure the importance of scientific research, we discover that its contribution consists not only in finding answers to a certain problem, but also in the set of new questions that arise in the process. These are the new paths...

As an artist, I find this book on diaphragmatic hypertonia in lyric singers a true encouragement. To be able to count on the scientific support of a serious research on a subject that has never been investigated before is a unique privilege and has its historical contribution. As lyric singing is a highly specialized activity that involves the whole body, as well as psycho-emotional aspects, it is extremely necessary to promote new research in this area, and the interdisciplinary contribution between scientists and performers is indispensable. This is the greatest differential of this book! Tati Helene's deep theoretical and practical knowledge of the process of lyric singing, combined with her background as a physical therapist, makes her detailed writing assertive and accessible, speaking directly to the performer who experiences these mechanisms in their daily lives, without having to abandon the technical terms that are used by health professionals. The book awakens in the performer reader an interest in monitoring diaphragmatic tone and can provide didactic insights for both the technical improvement of professional soloists and the singing teacher.

From the point of view of an enthusiast of technological innovations, I see in this research a real treasure trove for the development of artificial intelligence software in the medical field. I consider the author's description of the biomechanics of lyrical singing very useful for neuroplasticity studies, and I believe that the crossing of the information presented with other research in the area can contribute not only to a deeper study of the singer's pathologies, but also to the development of treatments for other respiratory diseases.

I strongly recommend this reading to fellow singers, singing teachers, speech therapists, physiotherapists, and neuroscientists, confident that the questions raised, still unanswered, may open paths for the future of lyrical art, medical science, and for a greater knowledge of this wonderful machine that is the human brain.

Elisabete Almeida, lyric singer

Introduction

Despite popular belief in an innate facility for singing, the reality is that a professional lyric singer trains not only his phonatory apparatus, but his whole body to be able to produce certain sounds. Their training routine and life is so intense and rigorous[1]that we can compare it to that of high performance athletes[2]. Both areas of performance involve training and bodily demands at the limit of what the human body can achieve, which is why Quarrier has already referred to all performance artists as athletes, and to musicians as music athletes in 1993 [3]. Because of this, we will hereafter refer to lyric artists as **voice athletes,** [4]and their specific technical movements as **artistic gestures**, in equivalence to the term **sportive gestures** we use when dealing with sport activity.

Since the creation of opera in the 17th century to the present day, many changes have occurred, both in terms of the artistic gestures used by voice athletes, the expressive skills required, and the length of career expected of a professional singer today.

Currently, the didactic activity of this art is based more on anatomy than on the original empiricism and vocal pedagogy has had great advances in the last decade. In the last decade, vocal pedagogy has made great advances. Otorhinolaryngologists and speech therapists have also started to search for technical improvement in the professional singing voice, [5]with the objective of providing singing teachers, professional

---

[1] Miller R. The Structure of Singing. USA: Schirmer; 1996. 372 p.
[2] Dick RW, Berning JR, Dawson W, Ginsburg RD, Miller C, Shybut GT. Athletes and the Arts - The Role of Sports Medicine in the Performing Arts. Current Sports Medicine Reports. 2013.
[3] Quarrier NF. Performing Arts Medicine: The Musical Athlete. Journal of Orthopedic & SportsPhysical Therapy. 1993;17(2).
[4] Helene T. Atletas da Voz - Manual para o Cantor Lírico. Porto Alegre: Editora Simplíssimo; 2020.
[5] David M. The New Voice Pedagogy. 2nd ed. USA: Scarecrow Press, Inc. 5882 positions. (Digital Edition).

singers and students with better conditions to prevent and treat the deleterious effects of this artistic practice on the phonation system.

It is known today that voice athletes alter the normal coordination of the thoracic cage and the abdomen during singing, with the probable purpose of avoiding the return of the diaphragm to the relaxed position, thus maintaining the ribs elevated, which generates a specific subglottic pressure[6], necessary for an efficient vocal production, by exerting considerable influence on the pressure level of the sound, on the fundamental frequency and on the resonances of the vocal apparatus[789]. The diaphragm, being the main muscle of respiration, in lyrical singing, is the primary muscle of the artistic gestures for sound production, [10]participating in inspiration, which is its physiological movement, [11]and in expiration, during phonation[12]. In the first chapters we will study these gestures in more depth.

This great demand and alteration in the coordination suffered by the respiratory muscles of a lyrical singer has raised the question whether, after years of professional career, alterations in mobility and tonicity can be created in the diaphragm of these voice athletes. Woodring and Bogner in 1998 already presented a case study in which they observed a high

---

[6] Salomoni S, van den Hoorn W, Hodges P. Breathing and Singing: Objective Characterization of Breathing Patterns in Classical Singers. PLoS ONE. 2016;11(5):1–18.

[7] Leanderson R, Sundberg J, von Euler C. Breathing muscle activity and subglottal pressure dynamics in singing and speech. Journal of Voice. 1987;1(3)(Raven Press, Ltd.):258-61.

[8] McAllister A, Sundberg J. Data on subglottal pressure and SPL at varied vocal loudness and pitch in 8 - to 11 -year-old children. Journal of Voice. 1998;12(2)(Singular Publishing Group, Inc.):166-74.

[9] Sundberg J, Elliot N, Gramming P, Nord L. Short-term variation of subglottal pressure for expressive purposes in singing and stage speech: a preliminary investigation. Journal of Voice. 1993;7(3)(Raven Press, Ltd.):227-34.

[10] Malde M. The Singer's Breath. In: What every singer needs to know about the body. 2nd ed USA: Plural Publishing Inc; 2013. p. 251.

[11] Rus MM. Manual de Fisioterapia Respiratoria. 2nd ed. Spain: Ediciones Ergon; 2003. 139 p.

[12] Leanderson R, Sundberg J, von Euler C. Role of diaphragmatic activity during singing: a study of transdiaphragmatic pressures. American Physiological Society. 1987;62:259-70.

diaphragmatic hypertrophy in a professional lyric singer, having the thickness of this muscle, evaluated via computed tomography, largely passed the maximum limit of normality. [13].

In the chapter on the evaluation of diaphragmatic tone and mobility, we propose a form of manual evaluation of this muscle, which is very accessible for clinical application in the office, as well as in a self-assessment for the athlete's own self-reference.

The most commonly used methods for assessing the strength of the respiratory muscles are the measurement of maximal respiratory pressures by manovacuometry, diaphragmatic ultrasonography, the sniff test, and also manual assessment[14]. We prefer manual assessment for its clinical practicality, since its use does not depend on any special equipment. The main authors to describe the manual evaluation of the diaphragm were the Argentinian A. Cuello in 1980 and, with G. Cuello and the Brazilian E. Aquino, in 2013; the Spanish T. Rial and P. Pinsach in 2015 and the Italians Bordoni, Morelli, Morabito and Sacconi in 2016 and 2017. Cuello addresses manual assessment with the purpose of measuring diaphragmatic and intercostal forces in the clinical use of respiratory physiotherapy, that is, with a look for diaphragmatic deficiency and/or desynchrony or other changes arising from respiratory pathologies [1516]. Rial and Pinsach describe how manual evaluation of the diaphragm can be done by a therapist or on oneself, addressing mainly the evaluation of hypertonic degrees of diaphragm that are usually more present in

[13] Woodring JH, Bognar B. Muscular Hypertrophy of the Left Diaphragmatic Crus: An Unusual Cause of a Paraspinal "Mass". Journal of Thoracic Imaging. 1998;13(Lippincott-Raven Publishers):144-5.
[14] Romani JCP, Miara N, Carradore MJK. Clinical Assessment of Respiratory Muscle Function in Adults: Review of the Literature. Cadernos da escola de Saúde. 2014;11(Faculdades Integradas do Brasil):1-19.

[15] Cuello AF. Kinesiologia pneumo cardiológica. Argentina: Editorial Sijka; 1980.
[16] Cuello AF, Aquim EE, Cuello GA. Ventilatory muscles - Biomotors of the respiratory pump - evaluation and treatment. São Paulo: Andreoli; 2013. 174 p.

athletes and indicating that its negative consequences include urinary incontinence, pelvic floor weakness, low back pain, prolapses, lumbar hernias, among others [17]. Bordoni et al, however, address in two studies the importance of manual evaluation of the diaphragm as an excellent tool for various physiotherapeutic approaches, from respiratory to postural evaluation, analysis of pain perception [18,19], among others, pointing out how much this procedure is essential for respiratory physiotherapists, manual therapists and GPR specialist [20].

The physiotherapist is responsible for analyzing the postural issues of the lyrical singer, as well as pain, tension, structural asymmetries, and any deleterious effect that affects the body systems due to his professional activity as a voice athlete[21]. Unfortunately, research on this particular group of voice athletes and their specificities with a physiotherapeutic view is practically non-existent. We only found the following works focused on physiotherapy and professional lyrical singing: Mauro Banfi, 2013, on postural alterations resulting from lyric singing observed in his clinical practice [22]and the Voice Massage® technique, described as a manual therapy technique aimed specifically at voice

[17] Rial T, Pinsach P. Ejercicios Hipopresivos - Mucho más que abdominales. Spain: La esfera de los libros; 2015. 3264 positions. (Digital Edition).

[18] Bordoni B, Marelli F, Morabito B, Sacconi B. Manual evaluation of the diaphragm muscle. International Journal of COPD. 2016;11(Dovepress):1949-56.

[19] Bordoni B, Marelli F, Morabito B, Sacconi B. Proposal for a New Manual Evaluation Scale for the Diaphragm Muscle: Manual Evaluation of the Diaphragm Scale - MED - Scale. International Journal of Complementary & Alternative Medicine. 2017;7(6)(MedCrave):1-7.

[20] Romani JCP, Miara N, Carradore MJK. Clinical Assessment of Respiratory Muscle Function in Adults: Review of the Literature. Cadernos da escola de Saúde. 2014;11(Faculdades Integradas do Brasil):1-19.

[21] Banfi M. Canto e Postura. Principi posturali ed osteopatici al servizio del cantante. Italy: Simplicissimus Book Farm srl.; 2013. 1341 positions. (Digital Edition)

[22] ditto

professionals [232425]; the study by Staes et al of 2011 on physiotherapy to optimize posture and vocal parameters, even though his study group is composed only of students and not lyric singing professionals [26]; and some studies not specifically physiotherapeutic but that seek to evaluate the musculoskeletal system in voice athletes [27282930313233343536]. This book was written with the purpose of filling this gap, opening the way for the production of more academic works about the activity of professional lyric singers.

[23] Koskinen L. Mitä Voice Massage on? [Internet]. Voice Massage. [cited February 3 2019].

[24] Leppänen K, Ilomäki I, Laukkanen AM. One-year follow-up study of self-evaluated effects of voice massage, voice training, and voice hygiene lecture in female teachers. Logoped Phoniatr Vocol. 2010 Apr;35(1):13-8.

[25] Leppänen K, Laukkanen AM, Ilomäki I, Vilkman E. A comparison of the effects of Voice Massage and voice hygiene lecture on self-reported vocal well-being and acoustic and perceptual speech parameters in female teachers. Folia Phoniatr Logop. 2009;61(4):227-38.

[26] Staes FF, Jansen L, Vilette A, Coveliers Y, Daniels K, Decoster W. Physical Therapy as a Means to Optimize Posture and Voice Parameters in Student Classical Singers: A Case Report. Journal of Voice. 2011;25(3):e91-101.

[27] Sataloff RT. Professional Singers: The Science and Art of Clinical Care. American Journal of Otolaryngology. 1981;2(3):251-66.

[28] Johnson G, Skinner M. The demands of professional opera singing on cranio-cervical posture. Eur Spine J. 2009;18(Springer):562-9.

[29] Amato R of CF. Analysis of the occurrence of thoraco-abdominal dyssynchronisms during the execution of respiratory strategy maneuvers by lyrical singers. In: XVIII Congresso da Associação Nacional de Pesquisa e Pós-Graduação (ANPPOM). Salvador; 2008. p. 368-71.

[30] Pettersen V, Westgaard RH. The activity patterns of neck muscles in professional classical singing. J Voice. 2005 Jun;19(2):238-51.

[31] Thorpe CW, Cala SJ, Chapman J, Davis PJ. Patterns of breath support in projection of the singing voice. J Voice. 2001 Mar;15(1):86-104.

[32] Watson, Alan. (2014). Breathing in Singing.

[33] Salomoni S, van den Hoorn W, Hodges P (2016) Breathing and Singing: Objective Characterization of Breathing Patterns in Classical Singers. PLoS ONE 11(5): e0155084.

[34] Wilson Arboleda BM, Frederick AL. Considerations for maintenance of postural alignment for voice production. J Voice. 2008 Jan;22(1):90-9.

[35] Peultier-Celli L, Audouin M, Beyaert C, Perrin P. Postural Control in Lyric Singers. J Voice. 2020 May 23:S0892-1997(20)30154-5.

[36] Scotto Di Carlo N. Cervical spine abnormalities in professional singers. Folia Phoniatr Logop. 1998;50(4):212-8.

1 - Respiratory biomechanics in lyrical singing

"The respiratory system is the power source in singing." [37]

Since the creation of opera in the 17th century until today, many changes have occurred, both in the artistic gestures used by singers and in the demands made on and the length of a professional singer's career.

In the beginning, the development of the artistic gestures of singing happened in an empirical way, from the effort to meet the main demands of the lyrical activity: that the artist has his voice heard throughout the theater, overlapping with the orchestra and the choir, and has a wide tessitura, vocal agility and vocal dynamics, among other attributes. Over the years, opera theaters have become larger and larger, orchestras have grown, their instruments have also evolved, increasing the volume produced and the *pitch has* also increased so that the instruments are brighter. With these changes, there have been increasing demands on the lyric singer's vocal and bodily effort[38]. After the Second World War, new technologies such as cinema, television and vinyl records, among others, directly influenced the way opera was performed, creating greater interpretative [39]and, consequently, physical demands on the singers.

In order to produce a sound that overcomes all these difficulties, the lyric singer needs to produce a specific subglottal pressure, and to do so he uses intense respiratory control. In this book we will deal only with artistic

---

[37] "The respiratory system is the power source of singing." (Free translation) STARK, James A. Bel canto: a history of vocal pedagogy. University of Toronto Press Incorporated. Toronto: 1999;

[38] PORTO, Henrique Marques. Opera at Risk - High Tuning in Orchestras is Harmful to Voices and Could Compromise Opera's Future . Opera Sempre website: 2012.

[39] ECHEVARRIA, Nestor. Historia de los Cantantes Líricos. Editorial Clarity. Buenos Aires: 2000;

gestures related to respiratory control, leaving out those related to the control of the phonation apparatus and its adjustments made for sound production.

The most important point of respiratory biomechanics in lyrical singing is the use of inspiratory muscles during expiration, which is where the sound production itself takes place.

In a normal physiological breathing we have, at the moment of inspiration, the participation of the diaphragm muscle and the external intercostals. In a forced inspiration the accessory respiratory muscles are also involved: the sternocleidomastoid, the scalenes (anterior, middle and posterior), the pectoralis minor and the serratus anterior. Normal expiration does not require the use of specific muscles, since the lungs' own elasticity is enough to return them to their original volume, whereas in a forced expiration the internal intercostals and the abdominal muscles (straight, transverse, and oblique) come into play. [40]

During lyric singing, inspiration can occur in three ways: the physiological, the forced[41] (as described above) and the mixed. The same singer can even change in the same performance between these three types of inspiration or prioritize only one of them, depending on the needs found in the pieces performed.

The mixed breathing, which was the only one not mentioned previously because it is very specific to singing, occurs by the need that the time of inspiration fits the musical tempo, which in most cases means that this should be faster than the time of a normal physiological inspiration, and to avoid a totally forced inspiration [42](the activation of too many accessory muscles, mainly the sternocleidomastoid and the

---

[40]Roussos C. Function and fatigue of respiratory muscles. Chest. 1985 Aug;88 (2 Suppl): 124S-132S.

[41] Pettersen V, Westgaard RH. The activity patterns of neck muscles in professional classical singing. J Voice. 2005 Jun;19(2):238-51.

[42] Thorpe CW, Cala SJ, Chapman J, Davis PJ. Patterns of breath support in projection of the singing voice. J Voice. 2001 Mar;15(1):86-104.

scalenes, interferes in the control of the vocal tract, especially in the laryngeal control necessary for singing, therefore, a totally forced inspiration is usually avoided). For this inspiration we use the resource of, in the previous expiration, using the maximum possible volume of residual air in the lungs, greatly reducing the intrapulmonary pressure, which will cause that at the moment of inspiration a good part of the necessary suction of air occurs quickly through the exchange of pressures with the external environment[43]. Another resource used to accelerate the inspiration process is to actively force the abdomen outwards (forcing the abdominal muscles to their relaxed position), accelerating the contraction and lowering of the diaphragm[44]. To avoid excessive activation of the sternocleidomastoid and scalene muscles, a greater participation of the other accessory respiratory muscles is also used: the pectoralis minor and the serratus anterior.

It is in the expiration used by voice athletes that the major differences with respect to muscle work and biomechanics appear, when compared to physiological breathing. During normal expiration there is closure of the costal gradil and relaxation and elevation of the diaphragm. In lyric singing, however, in order to control subglottal pressure in every musical phrase (which is usually much longer than the time of a common physiological expiration) this closure is delayed as much as possible, causing the diaphragm and external intercostal muscles to remain active in an eccentric way, thus slowing down as much as possible the movement of the costal grid[45]. Also for this same function, the accessory muscles serratus anterior and pectoralis minor are activated, although in

[43] Watson, Alan. (2014). Breathing in Singing.
[44] Chapman, J.L. (2006). Singing and teaching singing: a holistic approach to classical voice. San Diego, CA: Plural Publishing.
[45] Thorpe CW, Cala SJ, Chapman J, Davis PJ. Patterns of breath support in projection of the singing voice. J Voice. 2001 Mar;15(1):86-104.

some cases, at the beginning of expiration[46], the scalenes and the sternocleidomastoid are also activated. In this last case, for the same reason mentioned regarding the moment of inspiration, there will be a search for these muscles to relax, and in this case the relaxation is even more important, because this is the moment when phonation will occur. With the purpose of controlling and helping the expulsion of air during expiration, the abdominal muscles are well activated, but the internal intercostals are kept relaxed because they would promote the unwanted closure of the costal grid. Activation of the abdominal musculature increases intra-abdominal pressure which allows better control of the subglottic pressure necessary for phonation[47].

---

[46] Pettersen V, Westgaard RH. The activity patterns of neck muscles in professional classical singing. J Voice. 2005 Jun;19(2):238-51.

[47] Salomoni S, van den Hoorn W, Hodges P (2016) Breathing and Singing: Objective Characterization of Breathing Patterns in Classical Singers. PLoS ONE 11(5): e0155084.

Figure 1: Inspiration in lyric singing, with anterior projection of the abdomen.

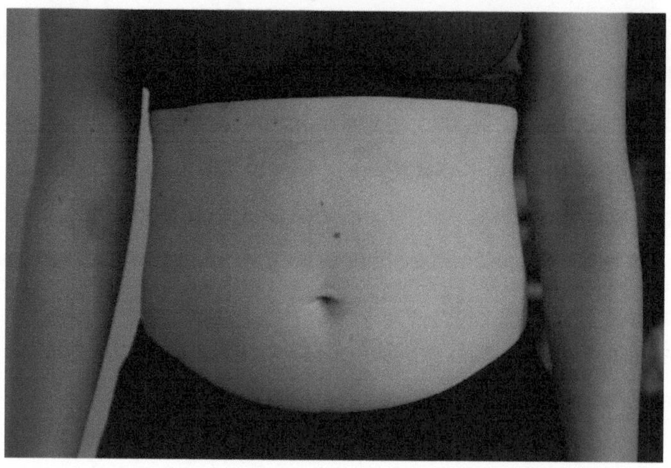

Figure 2: Expiration in lyric singing, with keeping the ribs open and the abdomen entering.

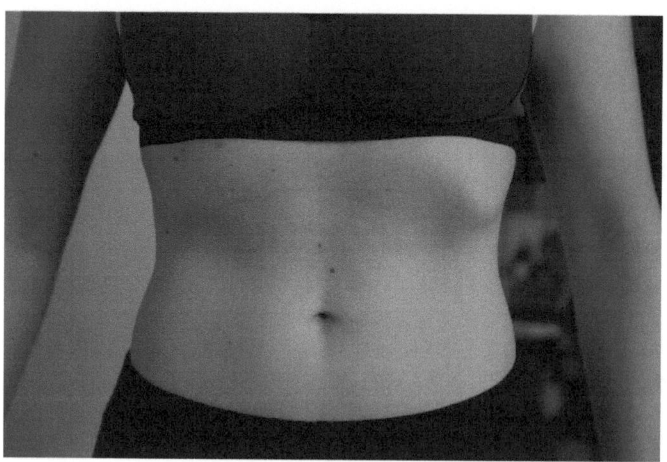

2 - Postural overload in lyrical singing

"A good posture is considered an optimum alignment of the body, with minimal energy requirements from the neuromuscular system without causing excessive strain on the various tissues. The effect of a change in one joint can have consequences anywhere along the kinetic chain. These changes can manifest in gait, joint load, neural function, endurance, strength, balance, muscle coordination, respiratory function, and ultimately the voice." [48]

There seems to be common agreement among voice science researchers that body posture is a very important point in controlling vocal production for lyric singers[49]. The posture most commonly described as ideal is one in which the feet are hip-width apart, slightly in contact and anchored on the ground, the knees are relaxed and uncrossed, the chest is high and open, the shoulders relaxed and the neck upright[50]. Different singing schools may, however, indicate variations from this ideal. The important thing is to be clear that the adoption of a more aligned posture interferes positively in vocal control and that it is one of the goals of the voice athlete to maintain this posture throughout the performance.

---

[48] "Good posture is considered when there is optimal alignment of the body, with minimal energy expenditure from the neuromuscular system, without causing excessive tension in the various tissues. The effect of a change in one joint can have consequences anywhere along the kinetic chain. These changes can manifest themselves in gait, joint loading, neural function, endurance, strength, balance, muscle coordination, respiratory function, and finally the voice." (free translation) - Cardoso R, Lumini-Oliveira J, Meneses RF. Associations between Posture, Voice, and Dysphonia: A Systematic Review. J Voice. 2019 Jan;33(1):124.e1-124.e12.

[49] Wilson Arboleda BM, Frederick AL. Considerations for maintenance of postural alignment for voice production. J Voice. 2008 Jan;22(1):90-9.

[50] Calais-Germain B, Germain F, Anatomie pour la voix. Comprendre et améliorer la dynamique de l'appareil vocal. Italie: Désiris; 2013.

The maintenance of posture during the performance of lyric singing is, therefore, another challenge to be managed by voice athletes, because their own artistic gestures (such as breathing movements and joints) interfere with postural control, significantly increasing the energy demand of the musculoskeletal system during the activity[51].

Other factors and conditions inherent to operatic performance also increase postural overload: besides the imbalances caused by the singing itself, voice actors are commonly subjected to other destabilizing factors, such as heavy costumes, which may have head ornaments and/or corsets, high heels, inclined stages, unstable scenery, and also the specific postural needs of each character[52].

To maintain posture and consequently good sound production, the lyric singer makes heavy demands on the musculoskeletal system. This, in turn, has a limited capacity to manage the excess of demand, usually causing muscle overload. As the years go by, the singer's body adapts to the high demands of artistic activity, undergoing transformations in its shape, its power and its reactivity, even when it is not active[53]. Di Carlo (1998), for example, has already observed in his study alterations in the cervical curvature of professional lyrical singers even at rest, probably due to the continuity of the execution of artistic gestures to control the vocal tract[54].

As we saw in the previous chapter, many of the muscles used for vocal control have a previous postural function, which significantly increases the demand on these muscles. The diaphragm, for example, is responsible for 80% of the respiratory work, but it also has other functions:

---

[51] Peultier-Celli L, Audouin M, Beyaert C, Perrin P. Postural Control in Lyric Singers. J Voice. 2020 May 23:S0892-1997(20)30154-5.
[52] Wilson Arboleda BM, Frederick AL. Considerations for maintenance of postural alignment for voice production. J Voice. 2008 Jan;22(1):90-9
[53] Banfi M. Canto e Postura. Principi posturali ed osteopatici al servizio del cantante. Italy: Simplicissimus Book Farm srl.; 2013. 1341 positions. (Digital Edition).
[54] Scotto Di Carlo N. Cervical spine abnormalities in professional singers. Folia Phoniatr Logop. 1998;50(4):212-8.

through the modulation of intra-abdominal pressure it participates in postural stabilization, helps in urination, defecation and childbirth, and is important for cardiac function and lymphatic flow[55].

Continuous overload on a muscle causes its hypertrophy. Woodring and Bognar (1998) have already written about the large hypertrophy found in the diaphragmatic muscle of a lyric singer[56] . The finding that most of the voice athletes in our study (detailed in the next chapter), showed diaphragmatic hypertonia, also points to this being another deleterious consequence of the poorly managed overload of the artistic practice of lyric singing for years[57].

---

[55] Kocjan J, Mariusz A, Bozena G-Z, Damian C, Mateusz R. Network of breathing. Multifunctional role of the diaphragm: a review. Advances in Respiratory Medicine. 2017;85(4):224-32.1.
[56] Woodring JH, Bognar B. Muscular Hypertrophy of the Left Diaphragmatic Crus: An Unusual Cause of a Paraspinal "Mass". Journal of Thoracic Imaging. 1998;13(Lippincott-Raven Publishers):144-5.
[57] Helene, Tati, Cristina Prota, and Angelica Alonso Castilho. "Manual evaluation of diaphragmatic mobility and tonicity in professional lyric singers and non-singers." *Fisioterapia Brasil* 21.5 (2020): 492-500.

3 - Diaphragmatic tonicity evaluation

The diaphragm tonicity evaluation proposed here can be performed in two ways: clinically, in which, in addition to tonicity, diaphragmatic mobility is evaluated, and by self-assessment, which allows the singer's own self-control and perception.

- Clinical Evaluation

It should be performed in three stages: Stage 1 and 2 - evaluation of diaphragmatic mobility, by the Manual Evaluation of the Diaphragm Scale (MED Scale)[58][59]and Stage 3 - evaluation of diaphragmatic tone according to the evaluation described by Rial and Pinsach, 2015 [60].

Stage 1 and 2 - The manual evaluation of the diaphragm must be done with the patient in dorsal decubitus, with knees bent and feet supported on the stretcher. To evaluate the mobility of the diaphragm the therapist should assess:

I. the costal movement during breathing, which consists of lateralization of the costal grid during inspiration with caudal direction and the opposite during expiration, with the examiner's hands gently resting on the sides of the costal borders [Figure 3];

---

[58] Bordoni B, Marelli F, Morabito B, Sacconi B. Manual evaluation of the diaphragm muscle. International Journal of COPD. 2016;11(Dovepress):1949-56.
[59] Bordoni B, Marelli F, Morabito B, Sacconi B. Proposal for a New Manual Evaluation Scale for the Diaphragm Muscle: Manual Evaluation of the Diaphragm Scale - MED - Scale. International Journal of Complementary & Alternative Medicine. 2017;7(6)(MedCrave):1-7.
[60] Rial T, Pinsach P. Ejercicios Hipopresivos - Mucho más que abdominales. Spain: La esfera de los libros; 2015. 3264 positions. (Digital Edition).

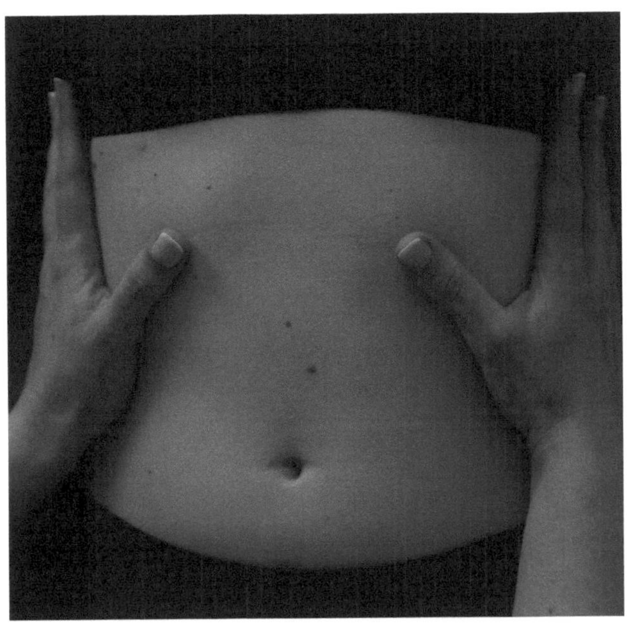

II. the diaphragmatic excursion during breathing. The diaphragm should lower during inspiration and raise during expiration, which will be gauged by the therapist with his hands positioned anterior to the rib borders, with the thumbs below the ribs at the lower costal margin and the other fingers gently resting on the upper ribs [61][Figure 4];

---

[61] Bordoni B, Marelli F, Morabito B, Sacconi B. Manual evaluation of the diaphragm muscle. International Journal of COPD. 2016;11(Dovepress):1949-56.

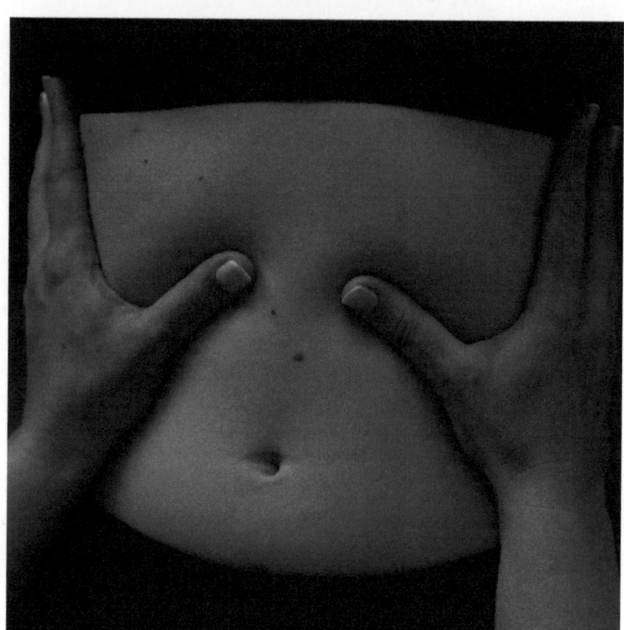

Figure 4: Evaluation of diaphragmatic excursion.

III. The MED Scale - Manual Evaluation of the Diaphragm Scale classifies each of the evaluation sites and their sides separately in 5 different gradations, as follows:

1. No movement restriction;
2. Slight restriction of movement;
3. Medium movement restriction;
4. Severe restriction of movement;
5. Motionless [62].

---

[62] Bordoni B, Marelli F, Morabito B, Sacconi B. Proposal for a New Manual Evaluation Scale for the Diaphragm Muscle: Manual Evaluation of the Diaphragm Scale - MED - Scale. International Journal of Complementary & Alternative Medicine. 2017;7(6)(MedCrave):1-7.

Step 3 - To assess the tone of the diaphragm, the therapist should place the thumb just below the costal edges and try to insert it under the ribs during the patient's expiration[63]. The assessment scale is of 3 possible gradations, these being:

1. *Normal*, when the examiner's fingers can penetrate one or two phalanges without any discomfort to the patient [Figure 5];
2. *Moderate hypertonia*, when the examiner has difficulty inserting the fingers and/or the patient feels discomfort [Figure 6];
3. *Severe hypertonia*, when the examiner's fingers cannot enter and/or the attempt causes discomfort to the patient [Figure 7][64].

The results are noted in a table specific for this evaluation, should be analyzed for diagnostic purposes, and archived for a comparative relationship after rebalancing approaches, for example [Table I].

---

[63] ditto

[64] Rial T, Pinsach P. Ejercicios Hipopresivos - Mucho más que abdominales. Spain: La esfera de los libros; 2015. 3264 positions. (Digital Edition).

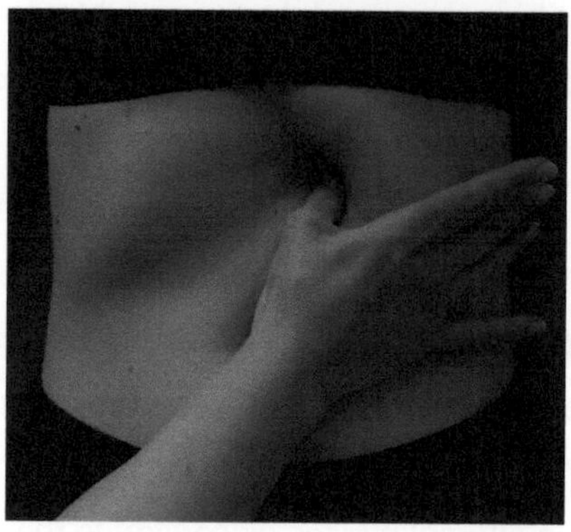

Figure 5: Normal gradation.

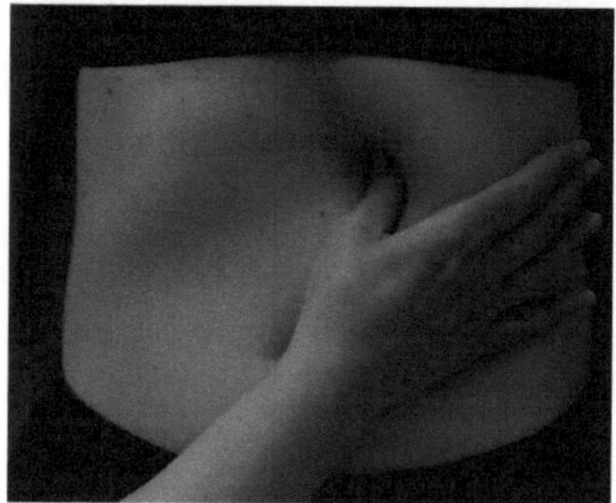

Figure 6: Moderate hypertonia gradation.

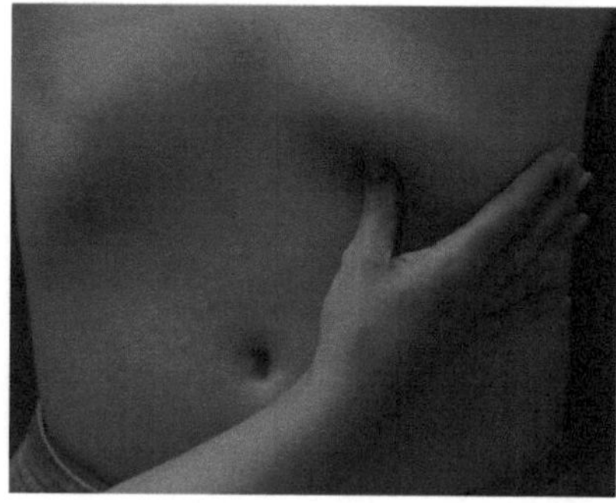

Figure 7. Gradation of severe hypertonia.

Table I. *Table used for clinical evaluation*

A) Diaphragmatic Mobility Assessment

Position	Law	Left
1 - Costal Movement		
2 - Diaphragm Excursion		

MED Scale:

1- No movement restriction
2 - Slight movement restriction
3 - Medium movement restriction
4 - Severe movement restriction
5 - No movement

B) Diaphragmatic Tonicity Evaluation

	Law	Left
Tonicity		

Degrees:

1 - Normal, when the evaluator's finger can enter from one to two phalanges without any discomfort to the patient
2 - Moderate hypertonia, when the examiner has difficulty introducing the finger and the patient feels discomfort
3 - Severe hypertonia, when the examiner's finger cannot enter and the attempt causes discomfort to the patient

- Self-assessment of tone

The self-assessment of diaphragmatic tonicity should be performed with the singer in dorsal decubitus, legs flexed and feet flat on the bed or floor. The singer should first feel with the four fingers of his hands (without the thumb) the region below his ribs [Figure 8]. The hands should be centered in relation to the body, with a distance of 3 to 4 fingers between the index fingers of each hand, and, as the singer exhales, he should try to introduce the fingers (especially the index finger) under his ribs.

Figure 8. Self-assessment of diaphragm tone.

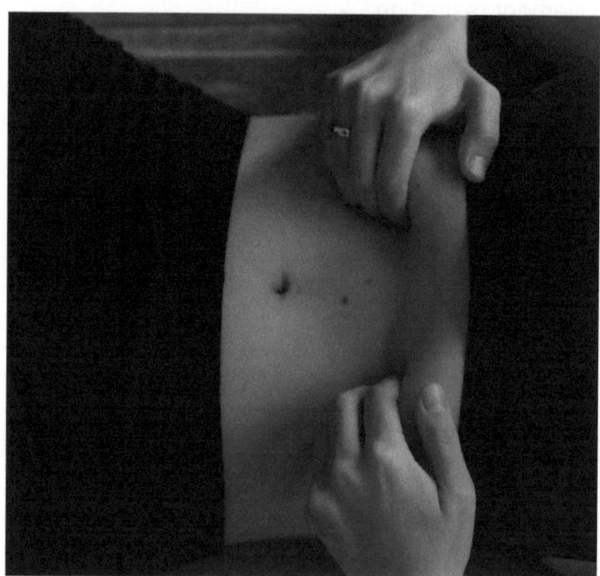

The rating scale is of 3 possible gradations, these being:

1. Normal, when the fingers achieve a penetration of one or two phalanges without any discomfort;
2. Moderate hypertonia, when there is difficulty introducing the fingers and/or discomfort;
3. Severe hypertonia, when the fingers cannot enter and/or the attempt causes discomfort[65].

If severe hypertonia on either side of the diaphragm or moderate hypertonia on both sides or only on the left side is observed, it is recommended that the singer consult a physical therapist.

- Cross-sectional controlled study

We did a controlled cross-sectional study to evaluate tonicity and diaphragmatic mobility in singers and non-singers in order to observe the differences between the groups[66].

The study was based on the norms of Resolution 466/12 of the National Health Council on research involving human beings and approved by the ethics committee of the São Judas Tadeu University under opinion number 3.327.706.

The participants, of both sexes, were divided into two groups:

---

[65] Rial T, Pinsach P. Ejercicios Hipopresivos - Mucho más que abdominales. Spain: La esfera de los libros; 2015. 3264 positions. (Digital Edition).
[66] Helene, Tati, Cristina Prota, and Angelica Alonso Castilho. "Manual evaluation of diaphragmatic mobility and tonicity in professional lyric singers and non-singers." *Fisioterapia Brasil* 21.5 (2020): 492-500.

I. professional lyric singers (G1)

II. Control group, composed of non-singers (CG).

The inclusion criteria were as follows: to be included in the G1 group, the participant should have been a professional lyric singer for at least 10 years; for the CG group, he or she should not exercise this activity, either as a professional or amateur, having a BMI and age similar to the G1 group participants. For both groups: they should not have had any disease that interferes with muscle tone and/or diaphragmatic mobility.

The exclusion criteria were as follows: for both groups, having had any disease or surgical intervention that altered muscle tone and/or diaphragmatic mobility, and for the CG group, not having age or BMI similar to the G1 participants, making it impossible to be paired with G1.

There were 54 participants in the study, 16 in G1 (Singers' Group) and 38 in the CG. One participant from G1 was excluded because he had physical alterations that could alter his tone or diaphragmatic mobility, and fourteen participants from the CG: six because they sang amateurishly, had studied singing formally or had some physical alteration that could alter their tone or diaphragmatic mobility, and eight because they did not resemble the G1 participants (four because they were over 60 years old, three because they were under 25 years old, and one because his BMI was 18.2 below normal). This left 15 participants in the singer group and 24 in the control group [Figure 9].

Figure 9. Flowchart of the sample selection process of professional lyric singers and control.

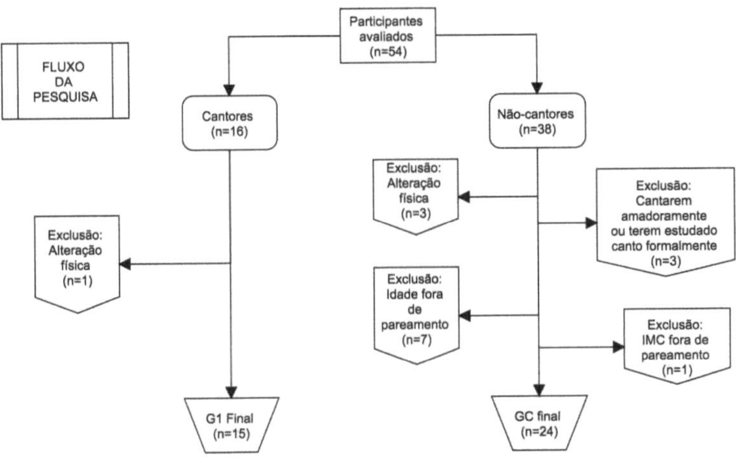

Table II describes the characterization of the sample divided by singer and control group, pointing out that there was no difference between them.

Table II. *Characterization of the sample of professional and control lyric singers.*

	Singers			Control			
	n	$_{Ma}$(dp)	**M**	**n**	$_{Ma}$(dp)	**M**	*p*
Age (years)	15	39.33 (6.4)	38	24	39.79 (7.69)	39	0.767
Age Fem (years)	7	40.42 (9.1)	37	13	38.53 (4.6)	38	0.955
Age Male (years)	8	38.37 (3.3)	38	11	27.73 (4.5)	41	
BMI (kg/m2)	15	27.64 (5.0)	24.7	24	25.76 (3.99)	25.35	0.275
BMI Fem (kg/m2)	7	27.52 (5.8)	24.7	13	24.76 (3.4)	24.3	0.694
BMI Male (kg/m2)	8	27.73 (4.5)	25.8	11	26.95 (4.3)	25.6	
Singing time (years)	15	20.4 (6.7)	20	-	-	-	-
Singing time Fem (years)	7	22.28 (9.2)	20	-	-	-	0.694
Singing time Male (years)	8	16.66 (2.1)	20	-	-	-	

Mann-Whitney U test / Legend: Fem- female; Masc - male; BMI - body mass index; $_{Ma}$- median; M - mean; dp - standard deviation

The manual evaluation of the diaphragm was performed by the same evaluator in both groups, without the evaluator's knowledge of the group to which each participant belonged. The procedure was performed as described above, after the participants accepted the TCLE and answered the questionnaire about health, lifestyle, and professional habits [Appendix]. The data were analyzed in the SPSS program version 20 and presented as mean, median, standard deviation, frequency, and percentage. The chi-square test was applied to the categorical variables. Initially the Shapiro- Wilk test was applied and as there was no normal distribution, for the comparison between the groups the Mann-Whitney test was applied and for the correlation of the demographic variables and mobility and diaphragmatic tonicity of the group of singers the Spearman correlation coefficient was used. For all statistical analyses, the significance level adopted was 5%.

When comparing the distribution of the manual evaluation of the diaphragm, we observed that the group of singers presented a significantly different distribution in relation to the bilateral tonicity of the diaphragm, with the individuals evaluated presenting greater hypertonicity in relation to the control group (Table III).

In the intra-group comparison of the singers' group in relation to gender there were no statistical differences (Table IV).

There was a moderate positive correlation between BMI and costal mobility D ($r = 0.605$; $p = 0.01$) and E ($r = 0.605$; $p = 0.01$); diaphragm excursion D ($r = 0.738$; p $p \leq 0.001$) and E($r = 0.,500$; $p = 0.05$) and diaphragm tone E ($r = 0.516$; $p = 0.04$) (Table V).

Table V. *Correlation between demographic variables (singing time, age and BMI) and the data collected (diaphragmatic mobility and tonicity) in the group of lyric singers*

	Singing Time r(p)	Age r(p)	BMI r(p)
Costal Mobility D	0.143(0.61)	0.321(0.24)	0.605(0.01)*
Costal Mobility E	0.143(0.61)	0.321(0.24)	0.605(0.01)*
Diaphragm excursion D	0.317(0.24)	0.42(0.11)	0.738(p≤0.001)*
Diaphragm excursion E	0.302(0.27)	0.45(0.09)	0.500(0.05)*
Tonicity and Diaphragm D	0.210(0.45)	0.08(0.75)	0.275(0.32)
Tonicity and Diaphragm E	0.05(0.84)	0.295(0.28)	0.516(0.04)*

Spearman's r $\qquad$ *$p \leq 0.05$

Legend: D - Right and E - Left

The moderate positive correlation between BMI and bilateral costal mobility, bilateral diaphragmatic excursion, and tonicity of the left diaphragm points us to changes in respiratory function with respect to weight gain, and does not correlate with singing time or the age of the individual. Obesity causes changes in the thoracic-abdominal region that lead to limited diaphragmatic mobility and costal movement, both of which are essential for good ventilatory mechanics[67]. Panizzi et al in 2004 have already pointed out in their study a tendency for decreased thoracic mobility in individuals with BMI above normal[68]. This finding may indicate that, for voice athletes, it is important to control their weight, so that there is no increase, beyond what the work activity itself already provides, of the chances of alterations in mobility, excursion, and tonicity of the diaphragm.

We conclude from this study that the artistic gestures used by professional lyric singers affect the tonicity of the diaphragm.

---

[67] Costa Melo L, da Silva MAM, Calles AC do N. Obesity and lung function: a systematic review. Einstein (São Paulo). 2014;12(1):120–5.

[68] Panizzi EA, Cordova FF, Pavan MP, Pamplona CM de A, Mozerle A, Kerkoski E. Mobilidade Torácica em indivíduos com peso corporal acima, no desável e abaixo do normal. In VIII Encontro Latino Americano de Iniciação Científica e IV Encontro Latino Americano de Pós-Graduação - Universidade do Vale do Paraíba; 2004. p. 467-71.

Table III- *Comparison between the groups of lyric singers and controls in the evaluation of the mobility and tonicity of the diaphragm*

		Singers		Control		
		F	(%)	F	%	χ2 (p)
Mobility costal D	Unrestricted	10	66.7	20	83.3	5.200 (0.07)
	Slight restriction	2	13.3	4	16.7	
	Medium Restriction	-	-	-	-	
	Severe restriction	-	-	-	-	
	Motionless	3	20%	-	-	
Mobility costal E	Unrestricted	10	66.7	19	79.2	5.283(0.07)
	Slight restriction	2	13.3	5	20.8	
	Medium Restriction	-	-	-	-	
	Severe restriction	-	-	-	-	
	Motionless	3	20	-	-	
Tour of Diaphragm D	Unrestricted	6	40	18	75	5.502(0.06)
	Slight restriction	8	53.3	6	25	
	Medium Restriction	-	-	-	-	
	Severe restriction	-	-	-	-	
	Motionless	1	6.7	-	-	
Tour of Diaphragm E	Unrestricted	8	53.3	20	83.3	5.468(0.141)
	Slight restriction	5	33.3	4	16.7	
	Medium Restriction	1	6.7	-	-	
	Severe restriction	-	-	-	-	
	Motionless	1	6.7	-	-	
Tonicity of the Diaphragm D	Normal	3	20	20	83.3	16.712(p≤0.001)*
	Moderate hypertonia	8	53.3	4	16.7	
	Severe hypertonia	4	26.7	-	-	
Tonicity of the Diaphragm E	Normal	6	40	17	70.8	6.613(.,03)*
	Moderate hypertonia	6	40	7	29.2	
	Severe hypertonia	3	20	-	-	

Chi-square test   *p≤0.05

Legend: D - Right, E - Left and F - Frequency

Table IV - *Comparison between genders within the group of lyric singers in the evaluation of the mobility and tonicity of the diaphragm*

		Female		Male		
		F	(%)	F	%	χ2 (p)
Mobility costal D	Unrestricted	6	85.7	4	50	3.348(0.18)
	Slight restriction	1	14.3	1	12.5	
	Medium Restriction	-	-	-	-	
	Severe restriction	-	-	-	-	
	Motionless	-	-	3	37.5	
Mobility costal E	Unrestricted	6	85.7	4	50	3.348(0.18)
	Slight restriction	1	14.3	1	12.5	
	Medium Restriction	-				
	Severe restriction	-				
	Motionless	-		3	37.5	
Tour of Diaphragm D	Unrestricted	3	42.9	3	37.5	0.938(0.62)
	Slight restriction	4	57.1	4	50	
	Medium Restriction	-	-	-	-	
	Severe restriction	-	-	-	-	
	Motionless	-	-	1	12.5	
Tour of Diaphragm E	Unrestricted	5	71.4	3	37.5	2.645(0.45)
	Slight restriction	2	28.6	3	37.5	
	Medium Restriction	-	-	1	12.5	
	Severe restriction	-	-	-	-	
	Motionless	-	-	1	12.5	
Tonicity of the Diaphragm D	Normal	1	14.3	2	25	0.268(0.87)
	Moderate hypertonia	4	57.1	4	50	
	Severe hypertonia	2	28.6	2	25	
Tonicity of the Diaphragm E	Normal	3	42,9	3	37,5	0.268(0.87)
	Moderate hypertonia	3	42.9	3	37.5	
	Severe hypertonia	1	14.3	2	25	

Chi-square test   *p≤0.05

Legend: D - Right, E - Left and F - Frequency

4 - The mobility issue

Hypertonicity is commonly accompanied by a loss of mobility, because the alteration in muscle tone makes it difficult to contract and fully extend the hypertonic muscle. The hypothesis of an interrelationship between decreased costal mobility and singing exercise, however, was not proven in this study. It is worth noting that the difference between the groups had a *p-value* very close to 0.05 and only in the group of singers, more specifically in the male participants of this group, were there distributions of costal mobility without movement, which was presented by 37.5% of the male participants.

These data draw our attention and lead us to question the limitations of this study, since they point to a trend toward decreased costal mobility in the group of voice athletes.

Our main limitation was the number of participants in the group of professional lyric singers. Because this is a very specific group, there is a difficulty in gathering a larger number of participants, which would allow us to eventually observe the changes in costal mobility with statistical relevance.

The results found, however, indicate that costal mobility in lyric singers should be frequently evaluated and, if alterations are found, treated by the responsible physiotherapist.

Another question arising from this difference in data between men and women, also of great importance during the physiotherapeutic treatment of voice athletes, is the difference in the behavior of respiratory dynamics between genders. Anatomical differences could explain this issue of lower mobility: women have a smaller radial dimension of the rib cage and a greater inclination of the ribs in relation to men, which promotes greater thoracic mobility during basal breathing[69]. In the case of males, therefore, due to the lower thoracic mobility, any change would be more noticeable.

These gender differences should also be evaluated in relation to fatigue and muscle overload. Schaeffer et al point to a greater perception of dyspnea in women than in men after physical activity, which comes from the existence of a greater neural respiratory motor drive to overcome the female dynamic mechanical restrictions[70]: with a smaller lung, women must breathe more often to supply the body with the oxygen needed for physical activity, increasing the work of the respiratory muscles, and therefore increasing their chances of getting into fatigue and accumulating overload.

New studies are essential to clarify this possibility of alteration in the costal mobility of voice athletes, particularly in males, with a larger number of participants, and to elucidate the differences in diaphragmatic overload between genders.

---

[69] MACHADO, Maria da Glória Rodrigues. Bases of respiratory physiotherapy: intensive therapy and rehabilitation. Rio de Janeiro: Guanabara Koogan, 2008. ISBN 9788527713658.
[70] Schaeffer, M.R., Mendonca, C.T., Levangie, M.C., Andersen, R.E., Taivassalo, T. and Jensen, D. (2014), Physiological mechanisms of sex differences in exertional dyspnoea: role of neural respiratory motor drive. Experimental Physiology, 99: 427-441.

5 - Harm of hypertonicity

The term muscle hypertonicity refers to an increase in muscle tone in general, which includes spasticity, rigidity, dystonia and contracture. For each of these conditions, the physiological mechanism causing hypertonicity will be different[71], but the deleterious consequences of its presence will nevertheless be the same. The fundamental difference will be in the various degrees of hypertonicity and, above all, in the treatment approaches.

In the previous chapters, and especially in the result of the cross-sectional clinical study, we have seen that the cause of diaphragmatic hypertonia in professional lyric singers is the specific use of the muscles over the years. We can therefore, in this case, consider hypertonicity as coming from a state of muscular semi-contraction, in which the diaphragm is kept in a lower position by increasing the degree of tension in its insertions[72].

The two diaphragmatic cruras insert the diaphragm posteriorly into the first 3 lumbar vertebrae (from L1 to L3)[73] . The cruras are joined by a fibrous median arcuate ligament. Excess tension from hypertonia can pull on these vertebrae causing excessive lordosis or curvature of the spine [74]with associated back pain[75] or postural imbalance. Changes such as hypertrophy or a lowered positioning of the median arcuate fibrous

---

[71] Mense S., Masi A.T. (2010) Increased Muscle Tone as a Cause of Muscle Pain. In: Mense S., Gerwin R. (eds) Muscle Pain: Understanding the Mechanisms. Springer, Berlin, Heidelberg.

[72] Urbanowicz, M. The dynamic diaphragm. Kinesiology Zone.

[73] NETTER, F. H. Atlas of Human Anatomy. 4 ed. Rio de Janeiro: Elsevier, 2008.

[74] Urbanowicz, M. The dynamic diaphragm. Kinesiology Zone.

[75] Barbosa, J.S., Almeida, L.P., Oliveira, M., Sacramento, M.D., Gomes, V.A., Petto, J., & Santos, A.C. (2020). Influence of the diaphragm muscle on postural control, proprioception and low back pain. Physiology of Exercise v18n4.

ligament can cause compression of the celiac artery, which can cause median arcuate ligament syndrome (which has epigastric pain and weight loss as its main symptoms) [76]or interfere with the function of the organs supplied by this artery: stomach, liver, duodenum, spleen and pancreas.

Figure 10. Anterior view of the diaphragm.

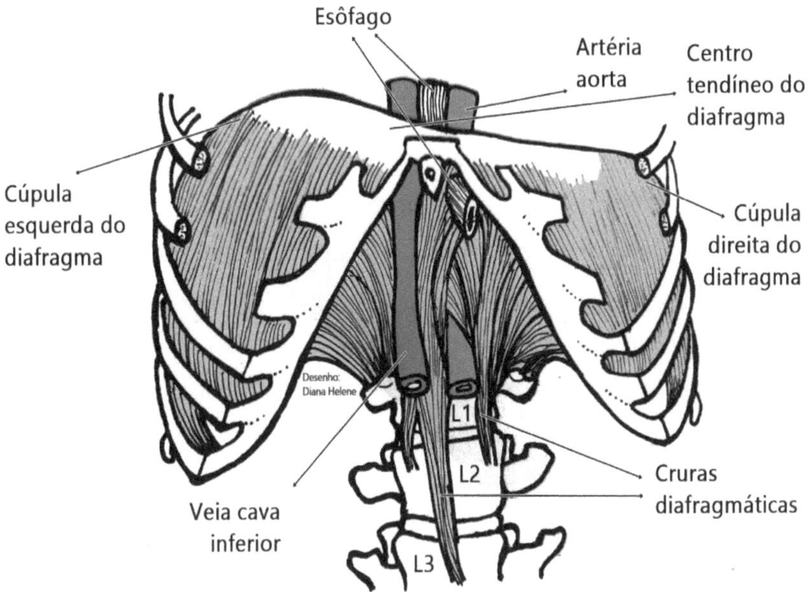

Excess tension can also interfere with the other insertions of the diaphragm. On the sternal side it inserts into the posterior surface of the xiphoid process and on the costal side into the internal surfaces of the lower costal cartilages and ribs 7-12, and tension may cause pain in these regions.

---

[76] Laura K. Nason, Christopher M. Walker, Michael F. McNeeley, Wanaporn Burivong, Corinne L. Fligner, and J. David Godwin. Imaging of the Diaphragm: Anatomy and Function. RadioGraphics 2012 32:2, E51-E70

Another possible dysfunction stemming from excessive tone in the diaphragm is a change in the functioning of the nerve and vascular structures that pass through it. The vagus and splanchnic nerves are responsible for communication between the intestines and the brain, sending constant feedbacks both afferent and efferent. If there is the presence of hypertonicity foci in the diaphragm (and consequently in the path to be taken by these electrical impulses) its capacity to transmit information can be altered, causing digestive problems [77]such as constipation, diarrhea, or dysbiosis, and/or dysfunctions in the autonomous nervous system, which interferes in stress management and in the body's rest cycles. The vascular alterations occur mainly in relation to the venous return and the lymphatic system, since the hypertonic state can hinder the fluid drainage system, which can cause the accumulation of fluids, with symptoms such as heavy legs, for example[78]

Rial and Pinsach in 2015 also suggest, as possible consequences of diaphragm hypertonia, prominent abdominal waist and pelvic floor changes, which may facilitate the appearance of hernias (abdominal or inguinal), prolapses and urinary incontinence [79], linked to a dysfunction in the management of intra-abdominal pressure (IAP). IAP is defined as the steady state pressure hidden within the abdominal cavity and results from the interaction between the abdominal wall, viscera, respiratory phases through movement of the diaphragm and pelvic floor[80] . Good IAP management occurs when all these structures move harmoniously and synchronously during the breathing process. A hypertonic diaphragm no

[77]Sardin, C. Back Pain, Anxiety, Digestive Disorder, Weak Pelvic Floor? Your Diaphragm Might be Guilty. Healthy by nature, 2019.
[78] ditto
[79] Rial T, Pinsach P. Ejercicios Hipopresivos - Mucho más que abdominales. Spain: La esfera de los libros; 2015. 3264 positions. (Digital Edition).

[80] Milanesi R, Caregnato RC. Intra-abdominal pressure: an integrative review. Einstein (Sao Paulo). 2016;14(3):423-430.

longer moves in this way and offers much greater resistance in the upper part of the abdominal cavity, thus increasing the pressure on the other structures and altering their functioning.

Changes in the diaphragm may also lead to hiatus hernia[81], one of the causes of Gastroesophageal Reflux Disease, which is more prevalent among professional singers than the average population according to Cammarota et al[82]. The authors report a statistically higher prevalence of heartburn, regurgitation, coughing and hoarseness in professional lyric singers than the population sample, with adjusted prevalence rates of 1.60 (95% confidence interval [CI], 1.32- 1.94), 1.81 (95% CI, 1.42-2.30), 1.40 (95% CI 1.18-1.67) and 2.45 (95% CI 1.97-4.04), respectively. The physiological explanation for these findings, whether or not there is a diagnosis of hiatus hernia, lies in the fact that in the lowered position of the diaphragm caused by hypertonia the esophageal sphincter muscles cannot close properly and allow reflux to occur[83].

Finally, osteopathic medicine currently refers to a model composed of 5 diaphragms: the cranial diaphragm (tentorium of the cerebellum), buccal diaphragm (tongue), high thoracic diaphragm (thoracic canyon), respiratory or low thoracic diaphragm, and pelvic diaphragm (pelvic floor). The authors defend that these diaphragms are deeply related to each other and that alterations in each one of them may interfere in the functioning of the others[84][85] . Thus, diagrammatic hypertonicity would have direct consequences on the other systems listed. This relationship

---

[81] Banfi M. Canto e Postura. Principi posturali ed osteopatici al servizio del cantante. Italy: Simplicissimus Book Farm srl.; 2013. 1341 positions. (Digital Edition).
[82] Cammarota G, Masala G, Cianci R, Palli D, Capaccio P, Schindler A, et al. Reflux symptoms in professional opera choristers. Gastroenterology. 2007;132(3):892-898.
[83] Urbanowicz, M. The dynamic diaphragm. Kinesiology Zone.

[84] Bordoni B. The Five Diaphragms in Osteopathic Manipulative Medicine: Neurological Relationships, Part 2. Cureus. 2020 Jun 20;12(6):e8713.
[85] Bordoni B. The Five Diaphragms in Osteopathic Manipulative Medicine: Neurological Relationships, Part 1. Cureus. 2020 Jun 19;12(6):e8697.

may also suggest an interference in the sound quality of the voice athlete, compromising its performance effectiveness. Unfortunately there are no studies with this approach yet, but Corrêa Machado et al point out an improvement in the production and sound quality of a sustained vowel after performing relaxation maneuvers and eccentric work of the diaphragm associated with an articulatory maneuver of the third cervical vertebra[86], indicating a possible relationship between diaphragmatic alterations and vocal production.

---

[86] Corrêa Machado, É., Fernandez Frigo, L., Anversa Bresolin, F., Lima, J., & Cielo, C. (2020). Immediate effects of cervical stimulation and diaphragmatic release on vocal production. *Physical Therapy in Movement, 33*, 1 - 7.

6 - Rebalancing and prevention approaches

In this chapter we will describe treatment approaches to hypertonicity of the diaphragm. It is fundamental, however, to point out that many of the deleterious consequences of this excess tonus can affect other structures and systems. We therefore recommend that once a patient is diagnosed with this condition, treatment should involve both the hypertonicity itself and the affected structure. If a pelvic floor dysfunction is observed, for example, both the diaphragm tonus and the pelvic floor dysfunction must be treated, because the latter, once installed, will not regress just by rebalancing the diaphragmatic tonus, requiring a two-pronged treatment.

As mentioned before, the treatment approaches for diaphragmatic hypertonicity, when one is seeking rebalance when for hypertonicity already configured or prevention so that it does not become established, are directly linked to its cause. In the case of voice athletes, the cause is in the specific demand of the artistic gestures of the profession itself, and these gestures cannot, therefore, be altered, so as not to compromise professional performance. The possible approaches for this group of artists are in the field of muscle compensation due to the high demand in the exercise of the profession, and for this reason can be used both for the objective of rebalancing and prevention.

With regard to muscle compensation, we have very little literature addressing this topic, and none specifically directed to voice athletes. We can fortunately, however, draw parallels with some studies on diaphragmatic hypertonia caused by exercise in general, and use metabolic and physiological concepts when thinking about possible approaches.

The manual evaluation of the diaphragm suggested above can be used clinically to assess diaphragmatic tone in voice athletes, and from this possible treatments for these alterations can be considered.

The abdominal hypopressive technique is defined as a postural and systemic technique[87] that causes a decrease in the tonicity of the diaphragm and as a consequence the decrease in IAP, activating by other physiological effects, different muscle groups that are antagonistic to the postural point of view of the diaphragm itself[88]. Caufriez, the creator of the technique, indicates that the systematic practice of the technique relaxes the diaphragm, normalizing its tone[89]. Rial and Pinsach also indicate the practice of the abdominal hypopressive technique as a form of approach in the treatment of diaphragmatic hypertonia caused by high demand in physical activities [90]. The *uddiyana bandha* movement of yoga and the abdominal vacum used by bodybuilders may also be a way to lengthen the diaphragm and thus interfere with its tone, but no studies were found that address the use of these techniques with respect to diaphragmatic tone.

Treatment approaches originally designed for diaphragmatic dysfunctions originating from other causes, such as those arising as a consequence of COPD, for example, excluding those of neurological origin,   are also feasible. The most common approaches found are manual therapy[91] , with the aim of releasing, relaxing and increasing the

[87] M. Caufriez, J.C. Fernández, R. Fanzel, T. Snoeck, Efectos de un programa de entrenamiento estructurado de Gimnasia Abdominal Hipopresiva sobre la estática vertebral cervical y dorsolumbar, Physical Therapy, Volume 28, Issue 4, 2006, Pages 205-216.

[88] Caufriez M, Fernández-Domínguez JC, Brynhildsvoll N. Estudio preliminar sobre la acción de la gimnasia hipopresiva en el tratamiento de la escoliosis idiopática. Enferm Clin. 2011 Nov-Dec;21(6):354-8. Spanish.

[89] Caufriez M. Gymnastique abdominale hypopressive. Caufriez: Bruxelles; 1997. p. 8-10.

[90] Rial T, Pinsach P. Ejercicios Hipopresivos - Mucho más que abdominales. Spain: La esfera de los libros; 2015. 3264 positions. (Digital Edition).

[91] Polastri M, Clini EM, Nava S, Ambrosino N. Manual Massage Therapy for Patients with COPD: A Scoping Review. Medicine (Kaunas). 2019 May 17;55(5):151.

mobility of the muscle; breathing exercises[92] , when the aim is to recover the strength of the respiratory muscles; and the practice of global physical activities[93] . In the case of voice athletes, due to the execution of their professional functions, it is deduced that there is no therapeutic reason for the application of respiratory strengthening or global physical activities, but that the manual therapy techniques can help in the objective of the release and tonic rebalancing of the diaphragm.

Braga et al suggest two manual therapy approaches aimed at releasing the diaphragm and increasing its mobility: diaphragm elevation and diaphragm relaxation. Diaphragm *elevation* consists of a technique of diaphragm stretching with support performed by the therapist and *diaphragm* relaxation, promotes greater relaxation of the diaphragm on its return during expiration with manual stimulation by the therapist [94].

González-Álvarez et al used the therapist-assisted *diaphragmatic stretching* technique to improve cervical extension, right and left cervical flexion, posterior chain flexibility and rib cage excursion at the xiphoid level[95].

Martinez-Hurtado et al indicate the *myofascial diaphragm release* technique as a way to improve the symptoms of patients with gastroesophageal reflux disease[96].

---

[92] Beaumont M, Forget P, Couturaud F, Reychler G. Effects of inspiratory muscle training in COPD patients: A systematic review and meta-analysis. Clin Respir J. 2018 Jul;12(7):2178-2188.

[93] Spruit MA, Pitta F, McAuley E, ZuWallack RL, Nici L. Pulmonary Rehabilitation and Physical Activity in Patients with Chronic Obstructive Pulmonary Disease. Am J Respir Crit Care Med. 2015 Oct 15;192(8):924-33.

[94] Braga, D. K. A. P., Marizeiro, D. F., Florêncio, A. C. L., Teles, M. D., Silva, Ítalo C., Santos-Júnior, F. F. U., & Campos, N. G. (2016). Manual therapy in diaphragm muscle: effect on respiratory muscle strength and chest mobility. *Manual Therapy, Posturology & Rehabilitation Journal, 1-5.*

[95] González-Álvarez, Francisco J et al. "Effects of diaphragm stretching on posterior chain muscle kinematics and rib cage and abdominal excursion: a randomized controlled trial." *Brazilian journal of physical therapy* vol. 20,5 405-411. 16 Jun. 2016.

[96] Martínez-Hurtado, I et al. "Effects of diaphragmatic myofascial release on gastroesophageal reflux disease: a preliminary randomized controlled trial." *Scientific reports* vol. 9,1 7273. 13 May. 2019,

The *Voice Massage®* technique, a manual therapy developed in Finland with the purpose of increasing the mobility of the rib cage when breathing and releasing the excessive tension in the various muscles used in voice production (speaking apparatus and respiratory muscles)[97], both for professional singers and other voice professionals, such as teachers and announcers, has also shown positive results in relation to the voice[98]. The technique also releases and lengthens the diaphragmatic muscles, but nothing in the studies published to date refers specifically to improved tonic rebalancing of the diaphragm.

Some authors also suggest an increase in treatment efficacy when manual therapy is associated with abdominal hypopressive technique[99], with faster results[100]. In his study, Muralimohan points to the efficiency of myofascial release of the diaphragm associated with Yoga breathing exercises (unfortunately the *uddiyana bandha* is not part of the exercises proposed in the study) in improving diaphragmatic mobility[101], but without a control group to see if there is a difference with the application of separate or associated techniques.

---

[97] Leppänen K, Laukkanen AM, Ilomäki I, Vilkman E. A comparison of the effects of Voice Massage and voice hygiene lecture on self-reported vocal well-being and acoustic and perceptual speech parameters in female teachers. Folia Phoniatr Logop. 2009;61(4):227-38. doi: 10.1159/000228000.

[98] Leppänen K, Ilomäki I, Laukkanen AM. One-year follow-up study of self-evaluated effects of voice massage, voice training, and voice hygiene lecture in female teachers. Logoped Phoniatr Vocol. 2010 Apr;35(1):13-8.

[99] Silveira TLR, Pontes RB. Hypopressive technique for subcostal line reduction in women: original article [Internet] [Article (Graduação em Fisioterapia)]. [Fortaleza]: universidade Federal do Ceará; 2019 [cited February 3, 2020].

[100] Bellido-Fernández L, Jiménez-Rejano JJ, Chillón-Martínez R, Gómez-Benítez MA, De-La-Casa-Almeida M, Rebollo-Salas M. Effectiveness of Massage Therapy and Abdominal Hypopressive Gymnastics in Nonspecific Chronic Low Back Pain: A Randomized Controlled Pilot Study. Evid Based Complement Alternat Med. 2018 Feb 22;2018:3684194.

[101] Muralimohan, R (2019) *Effectiveness of Manual Diaphragmatic Release Technique along with Yogic Breathing Practice on Improving Diaphragm Mobility, Inspiratory Capacity and Exercise Tolerance in COPD patients.* Masters thesis, Nandha College of Physiotherapy, Erode.

The approaches for rebalancing the diaphragmatic tone are also perfectly suited as strategies for prevention, and it is recommended that the professional lyrical singer be accompanied by a physiotherapist from the beginning of his vocal studies, in order to compensate for the great demands on the diaphragm and minimize postural imbalances[102]that may increase the demand on this muscle. Through this association it is possible to contribute to an evolution of the control of artistic gestures, effectively, but with less negative effect on the main muscle of respiration.

---

[102] Peultier-Celli L, Audouin M, Beyaert C, Perrin P. Postural Control in Lyric Singers. J Voice. 2020 May 23:S0892-1997(20)30154-5.

Final considerations

Voice athletes are a little-studied group of performing artists who need to be accompanied by a group of professionals from various specialties so that they can maintain their performance quality and deal with the overloads of the profession. The physiotherapist is an important ally in this multiprofessional team, because he can help from the beginning of the study with strategies for a better posture and evolution in the domain of artistic gestures, to the management of the overloads that come from the practice of lyric singing in the professional sphere, minimizing its deleterious consequences.

Bibliography

1. Miller R. The Structure of Singing. USA: Schirmer; 1996. 372 p.

2. Dick RW, Berning JR, Dawson W, Ginsburg RD, Miller C, Shybut GT. Athletes and the Arts - The Role of Sports Medicine in the Performing Arts. Current Sports Medicine Reports. 2013. DOI: https://doi.org/10.1249/jsr.0000000000000009 ;

3. Quarrier NF. Performing Arts Medicine: The Musical Athlete. Journal of Orthopedic & SportsPhysical Therapy. 1993;17(2). DOI: https://www.jospt.org/doi/10.2519/jospt.1993.17.2.90

4. Helene T. Atletas da Voz - Manual para o Cantor Lírico. Porto Alegre: Editora Simplíssimo; 2020. (Digital Edition).

5. David M. The New Voice Pedagogy. 2nd ed. USA: Scarecrow Press, Inc. 5882 positions. (Digital Edition).

6. Salomoni S, van den Hoorn W, Hodges P. Breathing and Singing: Objective Characterization of Breathing Patterns in Classical Singers. PLoS ONE. 2016;11(5):1–18. DOI: https://doi.org/10.1371/journal.pone.0155084

7. Leanderson R, Sundberg J, von Euler C. Breathing muscle activity and subglottal pressure dynamics in singing and speech. Journal of Voice. 1987;1(3)(Raven Press, Ltd.):258-61. DOI: https://doi.org/10.1016/S0892-1997(87)80009-7

8. McAllister A, Sundberg J. Data on subglottal pressure and SPL at varied vocal loudness and pitch in 8 - to 11 -year-old children. Journal of Voice. 1998;12(2)(Singular Publishing Group, Inc.):166-74. DOI: https://doi.org/10.1016/S0892-1997(98)80036-2

9. Sundberg J, Elliot N, Gramming P, Nord L. Short-term variation of subglottal pressure for expressive purposes in singing and stage speech: a preliminary investigation. Journal of Voice. 1993;7(3)(Raven Press, Ltd.):227-34. DOI: https://doi.org/10.1016/S0892-1997(05)80331-5

10. Malde M. The Singer's Breath. In: What every singer needs to know about the body. 2nd ed USA: Plural Publishing Inc; 2013. p. 251.

11. Rus MM. Manual de Fisioterapia Respiratoria. 2nd ed. Spain: Ediciones Ergon; 2003. 139 p.

12. Leanderson R, Sundberg J, von Euler C. Role of diaphragmatic activity during singing: a study of transdiaphragmatic pressures. American Physiological Society. 1987;62:259-70. DOI: https://doi.org/10.1152/jappl.1987.62.1.259

13. Woodring JH, Bognar B. Muscular Hypertrophy of the Left Diaphragmatic Crus: An Unusual Cause of a Paraspinal "Mass". Journal of Thoracic Imaging. 1998;13(Lippincott-Raven Publishers):144-5. DOI: https://doi.org/10.1097/00005382-199804000-00010

14. Romani JCP, Miara N, Carradore MJK. Clinical Assessment of Respiratory Muscle Function in Adults: Review of the Literature. Cadernos da escola de Saúde. 2014;11(Faculdades Integradas do Brasil):1-19. Available at: https://portaldeperiodicos.unibrasil.com.br/index.php/cadernossaude/article/view/2398

15. Bordoni B, Marelli F, Morabito B, Sacconi B. Manual evaluation of the diaphragm muscle. International Journal of COPD. 2016;11(Dovepress):1949-56. DOI: https://doi.org/10.2147/copd.s111634

16. Cuello AF. Kinesiologia neumo cardiológica. Argentina: Editorial Sijka; 1980.

17. Cuello AF, Aquim EE, Cuello GA. Ventilatory muscles - Biomotors of the respiratory pump - evaluation and treatment. São Paulo: Andreoli; 2013. 174 p.

18. Rial T, Pinsach P. Ejercicios Hipopresivos - Mucho más que abdominales. Spain: La esfera de los libros; 2015. 3264 positions. (Digital Edition).

19. Bordoni B, Marelli F, Morabito B, Sacconi B. Proposal for a New Manual Evaluation Scale for the Diaphragm Muscle: Manual Evaluation of the Diaphragm Scale - MED - Scale. International Journal of Complementary & Alternative Medicine. 2017;7(6)(MedCrave):1-7. DOI: https://doi.org/10.15406/ijcam.2017.07.00242

20. Banfi M. Canto e Postura. Principi posturali ed osteopatici al servizio del cantante. Italy: Simplicissimus Book Farm srl.; 2013. 1341 positions. (Digital Edition).

21. Koskinen L. Mitä Voice Massage on? [Internet]. Voice Massage. [cited February 3 2019]. Available from: https://www.voicemassage.fi/mitae-voice-massage-on

22. Staes FF, Jansen L, Vilette A, Coveliers Y, Daniels K, Decoster W. Physical Therapy as a Means to Optimize Posture and Voice Parameters in Student Classical Singers: A Case Report. Journal of Voice. 2011;25(3):e91-101. DOI: https://doi.org/10.1016/j.jvoice.2009.10.012

23. Sataloff RT. Professional Singers: The Science and Art of Clinical Care. American Journal of Otolaryngology. 1981;2(3):251-66. DOI: https://doi.org/10.1016/S0196-0709(81)80022-1

24.   Johnson G, Skinner M. The demands of professional opera singing on cranio-cervical posture. Eur Spine J. 2009;18(Springer):562-9.   DOI: https://doi.org/10.1007/s00586-009-0884-1

25.   Amato R of CF. Analysis of the occurrence of thoraco-abdominal dyssynchronisms during the execution of respiratory strategy maneuvers by lyrical singers. In: XVIII Congresso da Associação Nacional de Pesquisa e Pós-Graduação (ANPPOM). Salvador;   2008.   p.   368-71.   Available   at: https://www.academia.edu/40009017/An%C3%A1lise_da_ocorr%C3%AAncia_de_dessincronismos_t%C3%B3raco-abdominais_durante_a_execu%C3%A7%C3%A3o_de_manobras_de_estrat%C3%A9gia_respirat%C3%B3ria_por_cantoras_l%C3%ADricas

26.   Kocjan J, Mariusz A, Bozena G-Z, Damian C, Mateusz R. Network of breathing. Multifunctional role of the diaphragm: a review. Advances in Respiratory Medicine. 2017;85(4):224-32.1. DOI: https://doi.org/10.5603/arm.2017.0037

27.   Cammarota G, Masala G, Cianci R, Palli D, Capaccio P, Schindler A, et al. Reflux symptoms in professional opera choristers.   Gastroenterology.   2007;132(3):892-898.   DOI: https://doi.org/10.1053/j.gastro.2007.01.047

28.   Silveira TLR, Pontes RB. Hypopressive technique for subcostal line reduction in women: original article [Internet] [Article (Graduação em Fisioterapia)]. [Fortaleza]: universidade federal do Ceará;   2019   [cited   February   3,   2020].   Available   from: ~http://repositorio.ufc.br/handle/riufc/48748

29.   Costa Melo L, da Silva MAM, Calles AC do N. Obesity and lung function: a systematic review. Einstein (São Paulo). 2014;12(1):120–5.   DOI: http://dx.doi.org/10.1590/S1679-45082014RW2691

30.   Panizzi EA, Cordova FF, Pavan MP, Pamplona CM de A, Mozerle A, Kerkoski E. Mobilidade Torácica em indivíduos com peso corporal acima, no desável e abaixo do normal. In VIII Encontro Latino Americano de Iniciação Científica e IV Encontro Latino Americano de Pós-Graduação - Universidade do Vale do Paraíba;   2004.   p.   467-71.   Available   at: http://www.inicepg.univap.br/cd/INIC_2004/trabalhos/inic/pdf/IC4-65.pdf

31.   STARK, James. Bel Canto: A History of Vocal Pedagogy. 2nd ed. Canada: University of Toronto Press, 1999. (Digital Edition).

32.   PORTO, Henrique Marques. Opera at Risk - High Tuning in Orchestras is Harmful to Voices and May Compromise Opera's Future.   Opera   Sempre.   Available   at: < http://www.operasempre.com.br/2012/06/opera-em-risco-afinacao-alta-das.html>. Accessed 9 Feb. 2019.

33.   ECHEVARRIA, Nestor. Historia de los cantantes Liricos. Argentina: Editorial Claridad, 2000.

34.   Cardoso R, Lumini-Oliveira J, Meneses RF. Associations between Posture, Voice, and Dysphonia: A Systematic Review. J Voice.   2019   Jan;33(1):124.e1-124.e12.   doi: 10.1016/j.jvoice.2017.08.030

35.   Wilson Arboleda BM, Frederick AL. Considerations for maintenance of postural alignment for voice production. J Voice. 2008 Jan;22(1):90-9. doi: 10.1016/j.jvoice.2006.08.001

36.   Calais-Germain B, Germain F, Anatomie pour la voix. Comprendre et améliorer la dynamique de l'appareil vocal. Italie: Désiris; 2013.

37.   Peultier-Celli L, Audouin M, Beyaert C, Perrin P. Postural Control in Lyric Singers. J Voice. 2020 May 23:S0892-1997(20)30154-5. doi: 10.1016/j.jvoice.2020.04.019.

38.   Scotto Di Carlo N. Cervical spine abnormalities in professional singers. Folia Phoniatr Logop. 1998;50(4):212-8. doi: 10.1159/000021463.

39.   Chapman, J.L. (2006). Singing and teaching singing: a holistic approach to classical voice. San Diego, CA: Plural Publishing.

40.   Watson, Alan. (2014). Breathing in Singing. 10.1093/oxfordhb/9780199660773.013.10.

41.   Pettersen V, Westgaard RH. The activity patterns of neck muscles in professional classical singing. J Voice. 2005 Jun;19(2):238-51. doi: 10.1016/j.jvoice.2004.02.006.

42.   Salomoni S, van den Hoorn W, Hodges P (2016) Breathing and Singing: Objective Characterization of Breathing Patterns in Classical Singers. PLoS ONE 11(5): e0155084. https://doi.org/10.1371/journal.pone.0155084

43.   Roussos C. Function and fatigue of respiratory muscles. Chest. 1985 Aug;88(2 Suppl):124S-132S. doi: 10.1378/chest.88.2_supplement.124s.

44.   Mense S., Masi A.T. (2010) Increased Muscle Tone as a Cause of Muscle Pain. In: Mense S., Gerwin R. (eds) Muscle Pain: Understanding the Mechanisms. Springer, Berlin, Heidelberg. https://doi.org/10.1007/978-3-540-85021-2_6

45.   _ Urbanowicz, M. The dynamic diaphragm. Kinesiology Zone. https://kinesiologyzone.com/dynamic-diaphragm/

46.   NETTER, F. H. Atlas of Human Anatomy. 4 ed. Rio de Janeiro: Elsevier, 2008.

47.   Laura K. Nason, Christopher M. Walker, Michael F. McNeeley, Wanaporn Burivong, Corinne L. Fligner, and J. David Godwin. Imaging of the Diaphragm: Anatomy and Function. RadioGraphics 2012 32:2, E51-E70 https://doi.org/10.1148/rg.322115127

48.   Sardin, C. Back Pain, Anxiety, Digestive Disorder, Weak Pelvic Floor? Your Diaphragm Might be Guilty. Healthy by nature, 2019.   https://www.healthybynaturecalgary.ca/osteopath-calgary/diaphragm-affects-health

49.   Milanesi R, Caregnato RC. Intra-abdominal pressure: an integrative review. *Einstein (Sao Paulo).* 2016;14(3):423-430. doi:10.1590/S1679-45082016RW3088

50.   Bordoni B. The Five Diaphragms in Osteopathic Manipulative Medicine: Neurological Relationships, Part 2. Cureus. 2020 Jun 20;12(6):e8713. doi: 10.7759/cureus.8713.

51.   Bordoni B. The Five Diaphragms in Osteopathic Manipulative Medicine: Neurological Relationships, Part 1. Cureus. 2020 Jun 19;12(6):e8697. doi: 10.7759/cureus.8697.

52.   Barbosa, J.S., Almeida, L.P., Oliveira, M., Sacramento, M.D., Gomes, V.A., Petto, J., & Santos, A.C. (2020). Influence of the diaphragm muscle on postural control, proprioception and low back pain. Exercise Physiology v18n4

53.   Caufriez M. Gymnastique abdominale hypopressive. Caufriez: Bruxelles; 1997. p. 8-10.

54.   Caufriez M, Fernández-Domínguez JC, Brynhildsvoll N. Estudio preliminar sobre la acción de la gimnasia hipopresiva en el tratamiento de la escoliosis idiopática [Preliminary study on the action of hypopressive gymnastics in the treatment of idiopathic scoliosis]. Enferm Clin. 2011 Nov-Dec;21(6):354-8. Spanish. doi: 10.1016/j.enfcli.2011.06.003

55.   M. Caufriez, J.C. Fernández, R. Fanzel, T. Snoeck, Efectos de un programa de entrenamiento estructurado de Gimnasia Abdominal Hipopresiva sobre la estática vertebral cervical y dorsolumbar, Physical Therapy, Volume 28, Issue 4, 2006, Pages 205-216, https://doi.org/10.1016/S0211-5638(06)74048-2.

56.   Polastri M, Clini EM, Nava S, Ambrosino N. Manual Massage Therapy for Patients with COPD: A Scoping Review. Medicine (Kaunas). 2019 May 17;55(5):151. doi: 10.3390/medicine55050151

57.   Beaumont M, Forget P, Couturaud F, Reychler G. Effects of inspiratory muscle training in COPD patients: A systematic review and meta-analysis. Clin Respir J. 2018 Jul;12(7):2178-2188. doi: 10.1111/crj.12905. Epub 2018 May 23.

58.   Spruit MA, Pitta F, McAuley E, ZuWallack RL, Nici L. Pulmonary Rehabilitation and Physical Activity in Patients with Chronic Obstructive Pulmonary Disease. Am J Respir Crit Care Med. 2015 Oct 15;192(8):924-33. doi: 10.1164/rccm.201505-0929CI

59.   Braga, D. K. A. P., Marizeiro, D. F., Florêncio, A. C. L., Teles, M. D., Silva, Ítalo C., Santos-Júnior, F. F. U., & Campos, N. G. (2016). Manual therapy in diaphragm muscle: effect on respiratory muscle strength and chest mobility. *Manual Therapy, Posturology & Rehabilitation Journal, 1-5.* https://doi.org/10.17784/mtprehabjournal.2016.14.302

60.   González-Álvarez, Francisco J et al. "Effects of diaphragm stretching on posterior chain muscle kinematics and rib cage and abdominal excursion: a randomized controlled trial." *Brazilian journal of physical therapy* vol. 20,5 405-411. 16 Jun. 2016, doi:10.1590/bjpt-rbf.2014.0169

61.   Martínez-Hurtado, I et al. "Effects of diaphragmatic myofascial release on gastroesophageal reflux disease: a preliminary randomized controlled trial." *Scientific reports* vol. 9,1 7273. 13 May. 2019, doi:10.1038/s41598-019-43799-y

62.   Bellido-Fernández L, Jiménez-Rejano JJ, Chillón-Martínez R, Gómez-Benítez MA, De-La-Casa-Almeida M, Rebollo-Salas M. Effectiveness of Massage Therapy and Abdominal Hypopressive Gymnastics in Nonspecific Chronic Low Back Pain: A Randomized Controlled Pilot Study. Evid Based Complement Alternat Med. 2018 Feb 22;2018:3684194. doi: 10.1155/2018/3684194. Erratum in: Evid Based Complement Alternat Med. 2018 Sep 6;2018:3601984

63.   Leppänen K, Ilomäki I, Laukkanen AM. One-year follow-up study of self-evaluated effects of voice massage, voice training, and voice hygiene lecture in female teachers. Logoped Phoniatr Vocol. 2010 Apr;35(1):13-8. doi: 10.3109/14015430903552360

64.   Leppänen K, Laukkanen AM, Ilomäki I, Vilkman E. A comparison of the effects of Voice Massage and voice hygiene lecture on self-reported vocal well-being and acoustic and perceptual speech parameters in female teachers. Folia Phoniatr Logop. 2009;61(4):227-38. doi: 10.1159/000228000.

65.   MACHADO, Maria da Glória Rodrigues. Bases of respiratory physiotherapy: intensive therapy and rehabilitation. Rio de Janeiro: Guanabara Koogan, 2008. ISBN 9788527713658.

66.   Schaeffer, M.R., Mendonca, C.T., Levangie, M.C., Andersen, R.E., Taivassalo, T. and Jensen, D. (2014), Physiological mechanisms of sex differences in exertional dyspnoea: role of neural respiratory motor drive. Experimental Physiology, 99: 427-441. https://doi.org/10.1113/expphysiol.2013.074880

67.   Muralimohan, R (2019) *Effectiveness of Manual Diaphragmatic Release Technique along with Yogic Breathing Practice on Improving Diaphragm Mobility, Inspiratory Capacity and Exercise Tolerance in COPD patients.* Masters thesis, Nandha College of Physiotherapy, Erode.

68.   Corrêa Machado, É., Fernandez Frigo, L., Anversa Bresolin, F., Lima, J., & Cielo, C. (2020). Immediate effects of cervical stimulation and diaphragmatic release on vocal production. *Fisioterapia em Movimento (Physical Therapy in Movement), 33*, 1 - 7. doi:http://dx.doi.org/10.1590/1980-5918.033.AO37

Attachment

Participant Number: _________ Group: _________

Questionnaire on health, lifestyle and professional habits

Name: ____ **Idade**: _________

Profession:

____ **How many**

years have you held it? _____________

Weight:_________ **Height**:_________ **Sex**:_______ **Gender**: _________

Have you ever had a pregnancy?

[] no [] yes, how many? _____ [] I am pregnant at the moment

How were the births? _______________________________________

How long ago was the last one? _____________________

Do you practice any sport and/or physical activity?

[] yes   [] no [] I practiced but not anymore

Which one?

____

How often per week? _________________________________

How long have you practiced or practiced and how long have you

stopped?

____

How often do you sing every week?

[] every day [] 5 times [] 3 to 4 times [] 1 to 2 times   [] no singing

How many times a week do you drink?

[] every day [] 3 to 4 times [] 1 to 2 times []   only socially [] I don't drink

How many times a day do you smoke?

[] more than 5 times [] 3 to 4 times [] 1 to 2 times [] only socially [] do not

smoke

Do you use any other type of drugs?

[] no [] yes, how often? _____________________

Do you use daily medication?

[] no [] yes, which ones? _______________________________

Do you have any of the following diseases? (Check as many as

necessary)

[] hypertension   [] diabetes [   ] gastroesophageal reflux

[] cirrhosis []   gastritis [] cerebral palsy [   ] parkinsonism

[Thay-Sachs disease[] Down syndrome

[] muscular dystrophy   [] Prader-Willi syndrome [   ] trisomy 13

[] ligament laxity [] urinary incontinence

[low back pain (pain in the lower back)

Do you have any other chronic disease?

[] no [] yes, which? ____

Did you have any surgery?

[] no [] yes, which? _____________________ How long has it been?

____

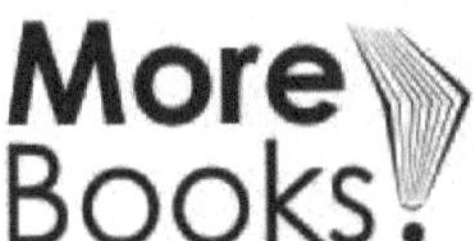

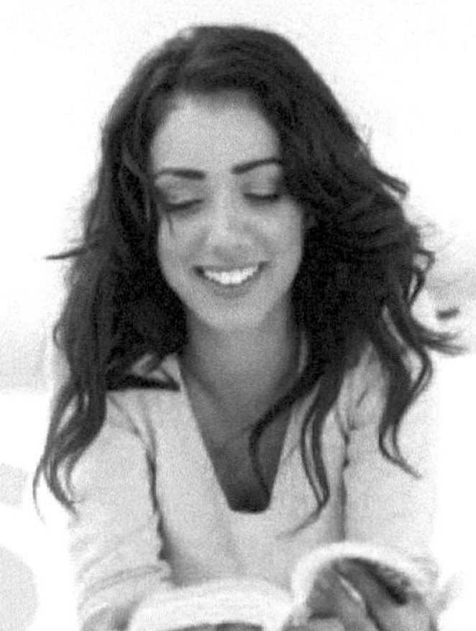

I want morebooks!

Buy your books fast and straightforward online - at one of world's fastest growing online book stores! Environmentally sound due to Print-on-Demand technologies.

Buy your books online at
www.morebooks.shop

Kaufen Sie Ihre Bücher schnell und unkompliziert online – auf einer der am schnellsten wachsenden Buchhandelsplattformen weltweit! Dank Print-On-Demand umwelt- und ressourcenschonend produzi ert.

Bücher schneller online kaufen
www.morebooks.shop

KS OmniScriptum Publishing
Brivibas gatve 197
LV-1039 Riga, Latvia
Telefax: +371 686 204 55

info@omniscriptum.com
www.omniscriptum.com

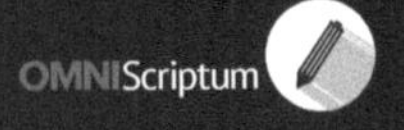

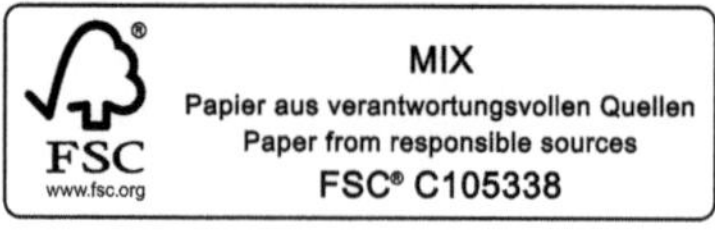

Printed by Books on Demand GmbH, Norderstedt / Germany